THANKS FO

MW01702890

MEDICATION LOG BOOK LARGE PRINT

DAILY MEDICATION TRACKER FOR SENIORS AND CAREGIVERS

All pages are presented **in large print for ease of reading,** with **ample space provided** for you to easily enter your information.

Each day is divided across two pages to ensure sufficient space for writing all of your details in large print.

This journal contains enough pages to **record your Medication for the entire year.**

The book also includes bonus pages for

- Personal Information,
- Doctor's Information
- Medical History
- Medical Visits /Tests / Checkups
- Medication / Supplement

Please **refer to the back pages** to find out how to obtain your BONUS EBOOK

brain & paint
BOOKS

Personal Information

Name:

Date of Birth:

Blood Group:

Weight:

Height:

Adress:

Mobile Phone:

Home Phone:

Email:

Doctor's Information

Name:

Medications:

Adress:

Emergency Contact

Email:

Mobile Phone:

Emergency Contact

Name:

Relationship:

Adress:

Email:

Mobile Phone:

Medical History

Diagnosed Health Conditions

Medical History

Diagnosed Health Conditions

Medical visits / tests / checkups

Date	Reason

Medical visits / tests / checkups

Doctor / lab	Notes

Medication / supplement...

Med / supp	Start / end Date

Medication / supplement...

Dose	Notes

MEDICATION LOG **DATE** ____________

MORNING		
MEDICATION	TIME	DOSE

AFTERNOON		
MEDICATION	TIME	DOSE

EVENING		
MEDICATION	TIME	DOSE

NOTES

MEDICATION LOG

DATE ____________________

MORNING		
MEDICATION	TIME	DOSE

AFTERNOON		
MEDICATION	TIME	DOSE

EVENING		
MEDICATION	TIME	DOSE

NOTES

MEDICATION LOG **DATE** ____________

MORNING		
MEDICATION	TIME	DOSE

AFTERNOON		
MEDICATION	TIME	DOSE

EVENING		
MEDICATION	TIME	DOSE

NOTES

MEDICATION LOG

DATE ______________________

MORNING		
MEDICATION	TIME	DOSE

AFTERNOON		
MEDICATION	TIME	DOSE

EVENING		
MEDICATION	TIME	DOSE

NOTES

MEDICATION LOG

DATE ______________________

MORNING		
MEDICATION	TIME	DOSE

AFTERNOON		
MEDICATION	TIME	DOSE

EVENING		
MEDICATION	TIME	DOSE

NOTES

MEDICATION LOG

DATE ____________________

MORNING		
MEDICATION	TIME	DOSE

AFTERNOON		
MEDICATION	TIME	DOSE

EVENING		
MEDICATION	TIME	DOSE

NOTES

MEDICATION LOG

DATE ____________________

MORNING		
MEDICATION	TIME	DOSE

AFTERNOON		
MEDICATION	TIME	DOSE

EVENING		
MEDICATION	TIME	DOSE

NOTES

MEDICATION LOG

DATE ______________

MORNING		
MEDICATION	TIME	DOSE

AFTERNOON		
MEDICATION	TIME	DOSE

EVENING		
MEDICATION	TIME	DOSE

NOTES

MEDICATION LOG

DATE ______________________

MORNING		
MEDICATION	TIME	DOSE

AFTERNOON		
MEDICATION	TIME	DOSE

EVENING		
MEDICATION	TIME	DOSE

NOTES

MEDICATION LOG

DATE ____________________

MORNING		
MEDICATION	TIME	DOSE

AFTERNOON		
MEDICATION	TIME	DOSE

EVENING

MEDICATION	TIME	DOSE

NOTES

MEDICATION LOG

DATE ______________

MORNING		
MEDICATION	TIME	DOSE

AFTERNOON		
MEDICATION	TIME	DOSE

EVENING		
MEDICATION	TIME	DOSE

NOTES

MEDICATION LOG

DATE ______

MORNING		
MEDICATION	TIME	DOSE

AFTERNOON		
MEDICATION	TIME	DOSE

EVENING		
MEDICATION	TIME	DOSE

NOTES

MEDICATION LOG

DATE ____________________

MORNING		
MEDICATION	TIME	DOSE

AFTERNOON		
MEDICATION	TIME	DOSE

EVENING		
MEDICATION	TIME	DOSE

NOTES

MEDICATION LOG

DATE ____________________

MORNING		
MEDICATION	TIME	DOSE

AFTERNOON		
MEDICATION	TIME	DOSE

EVENING		
MEDICATION	TIME	DOSE

NOTES

MEDICATION LOG

DATE ____________

MORNING		
MEDICATION	TIME	DOSE

AFTERNOON		
MEDICATION	TIME	DOSE

EVENING		
MEDICATION	TIME	DOSE

NOTES

MEDICATION LOG **DATE** ____________

MORNING		
MEDICATION	TIME	DOSE

AFTERNOON		
MEDICATION	TIME	DOSE

EVENING		
MEDICATION	TIME	DOSE

NOTES

MEDICATION LOG

DATE ____________________

MORNING		
MEDICATION	TIME	DOSE

AFTERNOON		
MEDICATION	TIME	DOSE

EVENING		
MEDICATION	TIME	DOSE

NOTES

MEDICATION LOG

DATE ____________

MORNING		
MEDICATION	TIME	DOSE

AFTERNOON		
MEDICATION	TIME	DOSE

EVENING		
MEDICATION	TIME	DOSE

NOTES

MEDICATION LOG **DATE** ____________________

MORNING		
MEDICATION	TIME	DOSE

AFTERNOON		
MEDICATION	TIME	DOSE

EVENING		
MEDICATION	TIME	DOSE

NOTES

MEDICATION LOG DATE ____________

MORNING		
MEDICATION	TIME	DOSE

AFTERNOON		
MEDICATION	TIME	DOSE

EVENING		
MEDICATION	TIME	DOSE

NOTES

MEDICATION LOG **DATE** ____________________

MORNING		
MEDICATION	TIME	DOSE

AFTERNOON		
MEDICATION	TIME	DOSE

EVENING

MEDICATION	TIME	DOSE

NOTES

MEDICATION LOG

DATE ____________________

MORNING		
MEDICATION	TIME	DOSE

AFTERNOON		
MEDICATION	TIME	DOSE

EVENING		
MEDICATION	TIME	DOSE

NOTES

MEDICATION LOG

DATE ____________

MORNING		
MEDICATION	TIME	DOSE

AFTERNOON		
MEDICATION	TIME	DOSE

EVENING		
MEDICATION	TIME	DOSE

NOTES

MEDICATION LOG

DATE ____________________

MORNING		
MEDICATION	TIME	DOSE

AFTERNOON		
MEDICATION	TIME	DOSE

EVENING		
MEDICATION	TIME	DOSE

NOTES

MEDICATION LOG

DATE ____________________

MORNING		
MEDICATION	TIME	DOSE

AFTERNOON		
MEDICATION	TIME	DOSE

EVENING		
MEDICATION	TIME	DOSE

NOTES

MEDICATION LOG DATE

MORNING		
MEDICATION	TIME	DOSE

AFTERNOON		
MEDICATION	TIME	DOSE

EVENING		
MEDICATION	TIME	DOSE

NOTES

MEDICATION LOG

DATE ____________________

MORNING		
MEDICATION	TIME	DOSE

AFTERNOON		
MEDICATION	TIME	DOSE

EVENING

MEDICATION	TIME	DOSE

NOTES

MEDICATION LOG

DATE ______________________

MORNING		
MEDICATION	TIME	DOSE

AFTERNOON		
MEDICATION	TIME	DOSE

EVENING		
MEDICATION	TIME	DOSE

NOTES

MEDICATION LOG **DATE** ____________

MORNING		
MEDICATION	TIME	DOSE

AFTERNOON		
MEDICATION	TIME	DOSE

EVENING		
MEDICATION	TIME	DOSE

NOTES

MEDICATION LOG

DATE ______________________

MORNING		
MEDICATION	TIME	DOSE

AFTERNOON		
MEDICATION	TIME	DOSE

EVENING		
MEDICATION	TIME	DOSE

NOTES

MEDICATION LOG

DATE ______________________

MORNING		
MEDICATION	TIME	DOSE

AFTERNOON		
MEDICATION	TIME	DOSE

EVENING		
MEDICATION	TIME	DOSE

NOTES

MEDICATION LOG

DATE ______________

MORNING		
MEDICATION	TIME	DOSE

AFTERNOON		
MEDICATION	TIME	DOSE

EVENING		
MEDICATION	TIME	DOSE

NOTES

MEDICATION LOG

DATE ______________

MORNING		
MEDICATION	TIME	DOSE

AFTERNOON		
MEDICATION	TIME	DOSE

EVENING		
MEDICATION	TIME	DOSE

NOTES

MEDICATION LOG

DATE ____________________

MORNING		
MEDICATION	TIME	DOSE

AFTERNOON		
MEDICATION	TIME	DOSE

EVENING		
MEDICATION	TIME	DOSE

NOTES

MEDICATION LOG

DATE ______________________

MORNING		
MEDICATION	TIME	DOSE

AFTERNOON		
MEDICATION	TIME	DOSE

EVENING		
MEDICATION	TIME	DOSE

NOTES

MEDICATION LOG

DATE ____________________

MORNING		
MEDICATION	TIME	DOSE

AFTERNOON		
MEDICATION	TIME	DOSE

EVENING		
MEDICATION	TIME	DOSE

NOTES

MEDICATION LOG

DATE ____________________

MORNING		
MEDICATION	TIME	DOSE

AFTERNOON		
MEDICATION	TIME	DOSE

EVENING		
MEDICATION	TIME	DOSE

NOTES

MEDICATION LOG

DATE ______________________

MORNING		
MEDICATION	TIME	DOSE

AFTERNOON		
MEDICATION	TIME	DOSE

EVENING

MEDICATION	TIME	DOSE

NOTES

MEDICATION LOG

DATE ____________________

MORNING		
MEDICATION	TIME	DOSE

AFTERNOON		
MEDICATION	TIME	DOSE

EVENING		
MEDICATION	TIME	DOSE

NOTES

MEDICATION LOG

DATE ____________________

MORNING		
MEDICATION	TIME	DOSE

AFTERNOON		
MEDICATION	TIME	DOSE

EVENING		
MEDICATION	TIME	DOSE

NOTES	

MEDICATION LOG

DATE ______________________

MORNING		
MEDICATION	TIME	DOSE

AFTERNOON		
MEDICATION	TIME	DOSE

EVENING		
MEDICATION	TIME	DOSE

NOTES

MEDICATION LOG

DATE ____________________

MORNING		
MEDICATION	TIME	DOSE

AFTERNOON		
MEDICATION	TIME	DOSE

EVENING		
MEDICATION	TIME	DOSE

NOTES

MEDICATION LOG

DATE ____________________

MORNING		
MEDICATION	TIME	DOSE

AFTERNOON		
MEDICATION	TIME	DOSE

EVENING		
MEDICATION	TIME	DOSE

NOTES

MEDICATION LOG

DATE ______________________

MORNING		
MEDICATION	TIME	DOSE

AFTERNOON		
MEDICATION	TIME	DOSE

EVENING		
MEDICATION	TIME	DOSE

NOTES

MEDICATION LOG

DATE ____________

MORNING		
MEDICATION	TIME	DOSE

AFTERNOON		
MEDICATION	TIME	DOSE

EVENING		
MEDICATION	TIME	DOSE

NOTES

MEDICATION LOG

DATE ____________________

MORNING		
MEDICATION	TIME	DOSE

AFTERNOON		
MEDICATION	TIME	DOSE

EVENING		
MEDICATION	TIME	DOSE

NOTES	

MEDICATION LOG

DATE ____________________

MORNING		
MEDICATION	TIME	DOSE

AFTERNOON		
MEDICATION	TIME	DOSE

EVENING		
MEDICATION	TIME	DOSE

NOTES

MEDICATION LOG

DATE ____________

MORNING		
MEDICATION	TIME	DOSE

AFTERNOON		
MEDICATION	TIME	DOSE

EVENING		
MEDICATION	TIME	DOSE

NOTES

MEDICATION LOG

DATE ____________________

MORNING		
MEDICATION	TIME	DOSE

AFTERNOON		
MEDICATION	TIME	DOSE

EVENING		
MEDICATION	TIME	DOSE

NOTES

MEDICATION LOG

DATE ______________

MORNING		
MEDICATION	TIME	DOSE

AFTERNOON		
MEDICATION	TIME	DOSE

EVENING		
MEDICATION	TIME	DOSE

NOTES	

MEDICATION LOG

DATE ____________

MORNING		
MEDICATION	TIME	DOSE

AFTERNOON		
MEDICATION	TIME	DOSE

EVENING		
MEDICATION	TIME	DOSE

NOTES

MEDICATION LOG **DATE** ____________________

MORNING		
MEDICATION	TIME	DOSE

AFTERNOON		
MEDICATION	TIME	DOSE

EVENING		
MEDICATION	TIME	DOSE

NOTES

Made in United States
Orlando, FL
05 July 2025

62665543R00066